MIGRAINE RELIEF REPORT

Ending Migraines Permanently with

Drug Free Biofunctional Process

Force Overload Cause of Inflammation Discovered

Corrective Biofunctional Process Ends Migraines

The Permanent Migraine Solution

Robert F. Mansueto, D.D.S.

Disclaimer

This book is not intended as medical advice. This book is intended to share the author's research, observations, and findings, as would an investigative journalist. This book is provided for informational and educational purposes. Please consult a licensed health care provider with any medical problems you may have. This book is not a substitute for professional health care. The statements in this book have not been evaluated by the FDA.

TABLE OF CONTENTS

ABOUT THE AUTHOR

Dr. Robert Mansueto is an implant surgeon, reconstructive dentist, scientist, and inventor who received his DDS degree at age 23, the youngest in the nation in 1976. He was accepted to doctoral school after 3 years of undergraduate studies at the University of Southern California where he studied biology, psychology, and physics. After graduating dental school, he served in the United States Navy Dental Corps at North Island Naval Air Station, San Diego Regional Dental center for several years, where he received advanced specialty and surgical training. He later joined a private practice in Coronado California where he pioneered early use of dental implants in the early1980's. He also invented and received FDA approval for a unique dental implant system in the 1990's and attained Fellow in the American Academy of Implant Dentistry, with some of his implant work having been published in the international Journal of Implant Dentistry.

After over 20 years in practice and engagement with other health care professionals and researchers inside the dental implant community, he discovered a biomechanical force overload cause and biofunctional corrective regimen that relieves the age-old malady of chronic migraines after he incidentally recognizing a corrective process and cause of migraines in one of his patients. He shared his discovery and findings with his sister-in-law dentist in practice with him and her osteopathic medical doctor husband, who together studied and analyzed this discovery, which Dr. Mansueto later described in detail including the underlying science of the underlying disorder that was incidentally discovered after a corrective process eliminated migraines in a group of 40 test patients. The detailed explanation of the discovery involved many different disciplines including physiology, mathematics, physics of force generation and force transfers, an area of strength for him with his educational background in implant dentistry as well as prior study of mathematics and physics that started at a very young age with tutoring from his father, a Navy pilot with a master's degree in mathematics and engineering. The corrective process Dr. Mansueto discovered, perfected, and described has since helped hundreds of patients in clinical trials and beyond.

His contributions and study helped to describe and perfect a process to resolve inflammation of traumatized tissues in the head and cranium and bring forth a long-term remedy for chronic headaches and migraines from his now proven force overload theory entitled DCFD-(Dento-Cranial Force Disorder). Contributors and participants to this effort also included other implant dentists, osteopathic medical practitioners, chiropractors, and a PhD in biomechanics. Without the contributions of this unique group of dental implant pioneers and other scientists, the groundbreaking findings and conclusions related to DCFD presented herein may not have been achieved.

To date, the findings presented in this initial release have helped hundreds of patients achieve permanent relief of chronic migraine pain. Dr. Mansueto is current director of World Migraine Relief Centers which may be visited at www.WorldMigraine.com along with leading an ongoing dental implant training and teaching program at American Dental Implant Center just inside the San Diego -Baja California Border.

PREFACE: THE MIGRAINE REPORT

This book was written to share monumental discoveries by a collaboration of doctors who discovered biofunctional corrective procedures that resolved migraine headaches. It started with a female dentist group member who volunteered to be an experimental patient for a new approach that altered biomechanical force mechanics in the jaws and head to see if it would help her chronic migraine pain. The following will discuss its success and implications for the future of migraine relief.

Migraine pain syndromes affect nearly a billion people worldwide. A true and understandable etiology with effective long-term solutions has remained elusive until the findings revealed in this publication. Herein, a collective mindset of many doctors across different professions reveal their discoveries and explain the biofunctional force overload disorder and cause that is both logical and understandable. When recognized, this disorder is 100% correctable.

Total costs of this disorder in North America alone have been estimated in the range of $100 billion dollars annually, not including the human suffering for which a price cannot be assigned. A viable solution to this age-old enigma that affects so many has been brought forth in this book, noting incidental discoveries of dental, chiropractic, and osteopathic practitioners that were found to predictably resolve migraine pain.

Repeat testing of procedures by a group of doctors from three different professions demonstrated consistent relief of migraine pain after biofunctional procedures were performed with an initial group of patients. This prompted the doctors to reverse engineer and analyze what each had done to produce this outcome and to exactly determine how the solution occurred.

As sometimes occurs in the fields of science, medicine, and the healing arts, incidental or accidental findings lead to new discoveries that can lead to new and improved treatments for people afflicted with disorders for which no solution had previously been identified. Such was the case when Dr. Alexander Fleming accidentally discovered penicillin mold growing in a petri dish in his lab in London in 1928. This led to tremendous benefits for millions and changed the landscape for the better in the medical world.

A similar incidental discovery occurred with a medical doctor's wife, a female dentist who suffered from chronic migraine headaches. She came to be the focal point of discovery of a physical force overload phenomenon that appears to be the cause of most migraines. In practice with her dentist brother-in-law, they experimented with a series of biofunctional corrective procedures that resolved her chronic migraines.

Earlier, that same biofunctional corrective process for migraines was postulated to be possible when this dentist and a chiropractor were working together on a mutual patient in the same time period, who reported that her migraine headaches had subsided during the course of their treatment. Similar corrective procedures were next used on the female dentist, who volunteered to be an experimental test patient for this conceptual approach. The results produced from a series of biofunctional corrections were total resolution of her migraine symptoms within a week. This led to cautious, bu optimistic investigation by four doctors, one being the patient who was married to a medical doctor, who also joined the collaborative that was formed. Needless to say, he was thrilled beyond words that his wife's migraines had seemingly disappeared.

Successful use of procedures utilized on this first experimental female dentist patient led to use on four more patients sourced from three different practices. The doctors wanted to see if they could successfully and predictably duplicate the process on more patients. All four of these patients were completely resolved their chronic migraine pain after the corrective procedures were administered.

Four doctors investigated and analyzed what had occurred, which led to recognition of a previously unknown biomechanical force overload phenomenon that they labeled Dento-Cranial Force Disorder, which was determined to be the etiology of migraines in one of their own, and then four others in a row. Group discussions and review of biosciences followed that focused on force generations in the Dento-Cranial Complex of muscles and hard tissues in the head. They were observed as generating compressive and pressure forces that transfer up into the head and cranium. It was further determined that when force generations exceed certain thresholds that traumatic inflammation and pain of migraine resulted.

The initial treatment regimen discovered was perfected over time and augmented with regenerative therapies suggested by the medical doctor that appeared to speed up resolution of symptoms and help patients return to normal lives again after years of migraine pain. Hundreds to date have had their lives drastically improved by freeing them of regular and recurring migraine episodes.

After seeing so many patients experience total relief of prior headache pain and "daily torture" within days after receiving a corrective biofunctional regimen, the collaboration of doctors was compelled to write this book to explain their findings and solutions. We have endeavored to explain the *why* and the *how,* so that the many people in need of migraine pain relief may hopefully learn of and understand the process, see the logic, and in turn, seek out this corrective care process that, while not widely known, is *non-surgical, drug free, and painless*.

Dento-Cranial Force Disorder or DCFD appears to be extremely common in the population as the likely cause of the majority of migraine syndromes in the population. This underlying causative disorder can further be predictably corrected once identified. Nowhere had any of the doctors in the group seen nor heard of any similar description of this etiology or corrective regimen. The doctors' collaborative grew to include other colleagues that all provided valuable input for this book. Without their help, conclusions and explanations would likely not have been found. We are thankful to them all for having contributed and being a part of the collaborative and collective mindset.

The authoring group realizes that oftentimes when something new and "too good to be true" comes along, there is often total disbelief, typically followed by criticism of varying degrees, all of which have already occurred. We all knew that we were not looking for this specifically at first, and that incidental findings led us down a path as if by "guided footsteps." We still wondered was this too good to be true? What would other doctors think about us for suggesting such an outrageous thing? We pondered this for quite some time. The realization set in as the days and weeks passed, with more patients reporting that their "headaches are gone, at least for now."

We all agreed on one thing: Biomechanical Force Overloads appear to be the underlying cause of most chronic migraines, a phenomenon not previously recognized, and certainly not widely known. Further to this, success rates of migraine pain relief observed after biofunctional corrective procedures were beyond significant according to any standard or interpretation of the scientific method. We also deemed findings and conclusions to be significant, as a direct cause and effect relationship was proven to exist. We believe these findings and biofunctional corrective procedures can potentially help millions of people who suffer from chronic headache pain, including those labeled Migraine, a word originally coined in the year 211 A.D. in Ancient Greece and translated into French.

After witnessing how a biofunctional treatment regimen improved the lives of many patients who suffered chronic migraine pain, we knew we had to share our findings and solutions with the public and try and help make the process available for the many people who also suffer, most having been told "there is no real solution" except drug therapy, shots, or in some cases nerve decompression surgery. Discovery of hidden biomechanically created force overloads as a cause of migraines involved chance occurrence at first, followed by a bit of trial and error. This ultimately led the group to refine a treatment regime that provides a rational and understandable basis to reduce or completely resolve traumatic inflammation and associated pain caused from biofunctional force overloads that are generated regularly in the Dento-Cranial Complex.

Successful results to date suggest strongly that DCFD appears to be the predominant etiology of the age-old migraine malady. No organic etiology had been identified in the past 2500 years. Practitioners and researchers alike have searched since the time of Hippocrates for an organic cause that could somehow be corrected but one just does not appear to exist. It appeared to the group that past researchers and clinicians had been looking in the wrong places all this time. Discoveries and realizations presented in this book provide logical and credible answers and solutions that occurred from the collaboration of doctors from three different professions working together, each bringing unique contributions and perspectives leading to conclusions that may not have otherwise occurred. The conclusions are based not only from success rates never before seen, but also on known science of biomechanics, physiology, physics, and mathematical principles that have been applied, along with demonstrable, logical, and duplicatable long-term solutions , defined as: "Resolution of head pain" for "Chronic Headache Syndrome", most often labeled as "Migraine".

An analogy used is of a small round tipped hammer being removed from a patient's hand who had been applying it to the side of their head several hundred times a day, making the comparison that after the hammer is taken away, pain, swelling and inflammation subside. It is exactly this type of force trauma that appears to be the overwhelming cause of migraine head pain that resolves after biofunctional corrections reduce traumatic physical force overloads. It all became so very logical to us and hopefully it will be to you the reader, as well.

The founding group, now expanded, is so very thankful to have been blessed with being able to present findings that have the potential to help the many who suffer chronic headache or migraine pain, beyond anything any of us had ever previously seen or heard of. We have attempted to explain our findings in layman's terms as much as possible, how this underlying force overload disorder was first identified, and how and why the corrective process discovered and refined works to resolve the underlying cause o trauma and inflammation that appears to be the overwhelming cause of most migraine pain. The underlying biofunctional force overload condition was seen to be extremely prevalent in the population yet has just not been recognized up until the present.

As we look back in history, and see when and where this all started, and the long path to where we are now, it is our sincere conviction that we have solved the age-old migraine enigma for the majority who suffer. It is further our mission to begin to help to serve the many who need long-term migraine relief. It is generally agreed today that an inflammatory process is indeed the cause of chronic headaches, including those labeled "Migraine". Now this previous enigma can be seen in a different light, using a new cognitive system, and a revolutionary way to resolve underlying traumatic inflammation that causes migraine pain, utilizing a corrective regimen that is non-surgical, drug free, and painless.

This book should be the single most important publication you read on this topic as it will enlighten you to this now understood logical source of trauma to the head and cranial structures that causes most migraine pain, and how it can be predictably corrected for long-term pain resolution. No logical cause or true remedy has been brought forth prior to this publication.

It is our sincere hope and prayer that our discovery and success to date helps bring forth relief for the many who suffer, as this corrective regime becomes more available. There are so many prior instructors, educators, and contributors to this project that it would be impossible to thank them all, from their sharing both concepts and clinical techniques as well as an impetus to always ask questions and look for solutions for human maladies that may be corrected, cured, or somehow made better.

DEDICATION:

This book is dedicated to the millions of people whose lives have been negatively impacted by the debilitating suffering of migraine pain disorders.

It is the sincere hope, prayer, and purpose of those who contributed to this publication that the information and corrective process presented herein provides a beacon of hope and healing for all your tomorrows to come.

INTRODUCTION:

This publication informs of a recent discovery of a biomechanical force overload disorder that emanates from the jaws and dental arches that was found to be a prevalent cause of migraine pain or chronic headaches. Additionally, an overview is given of a biofunctional corrective regimen of specialized dental and chiropractic procedures that was discovered, refined, and employed to correct these force overloads that relieved migraine pain in a trial group of 45 patients that had been suffering for three years or more. "Migraine" or Chronic, Repetitive Headache Syndrome affects approximately 15% of the population, nearly a billion people worldwide, with an overwhelming prevalence in women.

Incidental findings of significant reduction in migraine pain were first reported by a female patient who was undergoing dental reconstruction work while she was also seeing a chiropractor in the same time period. This prompted these two doctors to meet and discuss intriguing findings reported by this mutual patient. These doctors wanted to see if they could predictably duplicate the process in more patients.

The dentist knew that his sister-in-law, whom he was in practice with, also suffered migraines. He then spoke with her about trying similar procedures on her in an attempt to duplicate migraine pain relief reported by a previous patient. Dr. Dana, a female dentist, offered to be an "experimental patient" in hopes of obtaining migraine pain relief from a similar corrective process of dental alterations and chiropractic manipulations that provided relief in another patient. Dr. Dana was married to an osteopathic medical doctor[1] who

---

[1] Medical Doctor specializing in the musculoskeletal system, interconnected system of nerves, muscles, and bones combined with traditional medicine (osteopathic.org)

practiced nearby and who performed regular cranial manipulations on her that helped provide some migraine pain relief.

The same dental and chiropractic regimen used on a previous patient who reported migraine relief was performed on Dr. Dana over the next week. This led to drastic resolution of her migraine pain that was noticeable within two days. She recognized permanent relief after another week had passed.

This encouraging result led to a meeting of all four doctors, now including Dr. Dana and her medical doctor husband, to discuss and analyze what had occurred. A collaboration of doctors from three different professions was now underway from dental, medical, and chiropractic professions to investigate the intriguing findings of migraine relief now seen with two patients to date. All four doctors, one being the patient, each brought unique perspectives to the table to help analyze and draw conclusions of what had occurred to cause migraine pain relief for two patients in a row now. The two dentists were aware that specific alterations in dental bite patterns could cause changes in force magnitudes in the jaws that could be relatively quantified using mathematical formulas to generate mathematical conclusions that were not speculative. The group discussed using mathematical formulas of force mechanics to forces that were generated in the jaws and dental arches.

A force overload disorder was first suspected by the chiropractor as he had also been attempting to lessen symptoms in cranial areas from what he believed was some sort of trauma in the first female patient who reported migraine relief to her dentist. Mathematical conclusions observed in force formulas using muscle pressures and dental arch contacting areas helped the group to refine a regimen and standardize a protocol to use with the next group of patients they planned to test with this new promising treatment process based upon altering of force mechanics in the jaws and head structures.

Next, four additional female patients were gathered from these doctors' separate practices to further test and analyze their theory and findings to date. These patients were first seen by the two dentists in the group for initial evaluation of dental arch biomechanics and bite patterns suspected as being at the core of a force overload disorder. Dental bite patterns along with jaw and cranial bone alignments were significantly changed in both prior patients who in turn reported significant migraine pain relief after these alterations were made. Dr. Dana also related her own experience firsthand to these next few patients who volunteered to help evaluate a new and unknown process on the complex topic of migraine head pain that carried with it a historical label of "cause unknown".

The same biofunctional regimen of dental, chiropractic and osteopathic procedures were employed with this next group to reduce excess force loads and correct their vectors of transmission that were suspected of causing force overloads seen as the cause of migraine pain in the previous two patients. Relief of migraine pain was reported by these four patients within days. All four experienced complete resolution of migraine symptoms in the following week. These positive results fueled continued analysis to gain a better understanding of what had occurred.

After witnessing results in four more patients in a row, the initial group thought out loud: "Could we really have discovered the elusive cause of this age-old malady... and further How to fix it?" When we realized success rate for relieving chronic migraine episodes in five patients in a row now was virtually 100%, we were startled, amazed, and even a bit scared at first. We remained cautiously optimistic. The group continued to refine the corrective process during this time that ultimately led to what appears to be a game changer for the majority of people who suffer chronic migraines. The group expanded to include several more colleagues who contributed to the collective think tank that helped to describe epic findings of a biofunctiona force overload disorder that clearly appears to be the cause of most migraines.

The group now realized that this corrective regimen of specific dental and chiropractic procedures now being performed with purpose and intent, led to complete resolution of migraine pain in five patients in a row. This led the group to conclude that force overloads identified emanated from the jaw complex traveled upward and served as a source of trauma that was the cause of migraine head pain in all five patients to date who experienced drastic migraine pain relief after delivery of a biofunctional corrective process discovered just weeks prior.

This newly identified overload condition was labeled: <u>Dento-Cranial Force Disorder or DCFD</u>. A corrective regimen that was incidentally discovered to relieve migraine pain in dental patients undergoing reconstructive dental and chiropractic care was analyzed and refined using mathematics of force generations. This helped the doctors group see the magnitudes of forces that were suspected of being the underlying source of traumatic inflammation and migraine pain in all patients they had observed.

"Sterile Cranial Inflammation" has been extensively reported in medical literature as being associated with migraine pain. This collaboration of doctors appears to have connected the dots in this age-old malady to identify a source of physical force trauma that appears to be a common and most likely cause of cranial inflammation referred to in medical literature that has been reported to exist in patients suffering migraine headaches.

A series of corrective procedures of mainly dental and chiropractic alterations discovered and discussed in this book that has been used on hundreds of patients as of this writing, that instigated drastic or complete resolution of migraine pain symptoms after these biofunctional procedures were administered.

Analysis and testing by this group of an initial corrective process incidentally discovered that resolved migraine pain led to identification and description of a previously unrecognized source of physical force trauma that was shown to be the cause of migraine pain in hundreds of patients observed to date with this underlying disorder as all were relieved of their chronic head pain after receiving biofunctional corrective process presented in this publication.

Chronic migraine pain, which has previously carried the label of "unknown cause" now appears to have an identifiable, logical underlying cause and solution for the majority who suffer.

This previously unrecognized cause of migraines now termed <u>Dento-Cranial Force Disorder or DCFD, revealed in this publication, has been found to be a correctable disorder that when properly administered, led to long-term relief of migraine pain in all patients seen to date who exhibited this underlying condition.</u>

CHAPTER 1
DENTO-CRANIAL FORCE DISORDER

DCFD is a biomechanical generated force overload condition in the head and cranium identified by a group of doctors from three different professions that was discovered to be the cause of chronic migraine pain in several test groups of patients. A biofunctional corrective process focused on alteration of hard tissue contact areas in the jaws and cranial structures was incidentally discovered and refined that resolved migraine pain in patients by significantly altering force generation patterns and force transfers in the Dento-Cranial Complex.

This led to the recognition and description of this force overload phenomenon as a predominant cause of migraine pain, as the corrective regimen drastically relieved pain in all patients in test groups that exhibited this underlying disorder.

Traumatic forces overloads that comprise DCFD were identified after realization that alterations in dental arches and cranial bones lowered migraine symptoms. This relief of migraine pain repeatedly seen in patients after a biofunctional corrective regimen appeared to be a clear cause and effect of excess force loads generated in the Dento-Cranial Complex to migraine pain.

The incidental recognition of a process that produced migraine relief led to reverse engineering of the procedures performed during concurrent dental and chiropractic sessions. This reverse engineering by a multidisciplinary doctors' group led to recognition of traumatic force loads that are continuously generated from the jaws and dental arches and then transfer upward. These force generations and transfers were recognized to be excessive in patients who suffered chronic migraine pain.

These excess biomechanical forces were recognized as a source of physical force trauma in the head and cranium that repeatedly caused inflammation, heat generation, and pain of chronic migraines in all patients in an initial test group of forty-five patients. All forty-five patients experienced drastic or full relief within two weeks or less after a corrective regimen was completed.

The doctors' group was aware that force generations occur hundreds of times a day in the jaws when muscle contractions squeeze jaw bones and dental arches together which led to further analysis of compressive forces created in this area continuously. Force overloads generated from jaw closure cycles were seen to somehow initiate and transmit pressure forces up into the cranium that caused migraine pain in test groups observed. Further study led to recognition of specific force mechanics at play and the exact parameters that were altered during the course of treatments by dental and chiropractic means that led to relief of migraine pain.

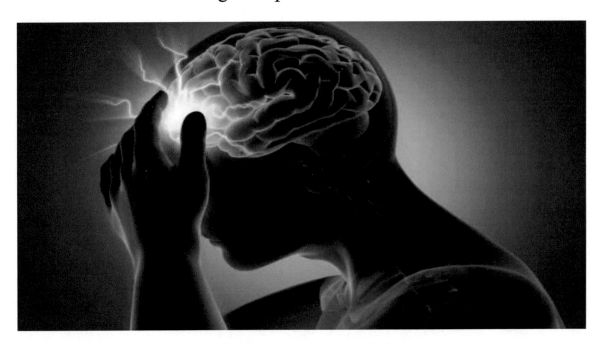

Excess Forces from Jaw Muscles turn into Painful Pressure Gradients

It was recognized that muscle pressure contractions and contact areas of hard tissues in the jaws and cranial bones combine to create force generations in the Dento-Cranial Complex that lead to DCFD and migraine pain in

18

individuals more susceptible to force overload induced inflammation, with females seen as being more susceptible than men to this force overload phenomenon.

Analysis of biomechanical factors involved in force generations in the jaw complex led to realization that pressure forces from muscle contractions, primarily from Temporalis and Masseter muscle groups pressing contract areas of hard tissues of dental arches and cranial bones together being the two primary factors that determine numerical conclusions using known mathematical formulas to calculate force magnitudes.

It was also determined that when either of these two parameters of muscle pressure or contact areas of hard tissues were adjusted downward, that lower force generations resulted. It was further seen that when force generations in the Dento-Cranial Complex were lowered in patients suffering chronic migraine pain, that rapid relief of migraine pain followed. Lowered force generations is exactly what occurs after Botox injections into facial-cranial muscle groups.

This discovery of this correlation of relief of migraine pain seen in patients after the biofunctional corrections led to a reverse engineering process using mathematics as a guide. Use of mathematics helped to reach the conclusion that excess force generations in the Dento-Cranial Complex leads to inflammation and head pain of migraine in susceptible patients with this underlying disorder. The correlation described above was seen in forty-five patients in a row leading to a logical conclusion that excess force generations fueled by powerful muscles of mastication are a source of physical trauma that led to inflammation and migraine pain experienced in all patient groups observed to date with this underlying condition. Further analysis of this biomechanical force etiology of migraine pain led to in depth analysis of compressive force loads generated during dental arch closure cycles that appear to translate or transform into pressure force gradients and travel

19

upward following a path of least resistance into the head and cranium causing traumatic inflammation and thus, head pain.

Discovery of these excess force loads that comprise DCFD were analyzed and quantified in clinical trials with several patient groups that led to a clear understanding of what causes them, how they progress to harmful excess force overloads that cause physical force trauma, and how these traumatic force overloads cause inflammation in the head that appear to be the prominent cause of migraine headaches in most people who suffer from this malady.

Use of Botox injections into Dento-Cranial muscle groups has been used to reduce muscle contractions in patients suffering from migraine pain episodes via partial paralysis of muscle fibers where Botox is injected, provided this investigating group a big clue, as Botox injections cause lowering of force generations in the Dento-Cranial Complex by reducing muscle contractions and their pressure generations. This observation of how Botox affects biomechanics in the Dento-Cranial complex that in turn reduces migraine episodes helped this group validate the force overload disorder now known as DCFD as causative of migraine pain. Incapacitating muscle fibers by inducing partial paralysis with Botox injections lowers pressure numerators used in mathematical formulas of force calculations. This same lowering of force generations can also occur by altering areas of contact in hard tissues attached to these same muscle groups when inserted into the same math formulas such as: P x A = F (Pressure x Area = Force) and others that were used to quantify force magnitudes generated. This direct correlation of lowered force generations in the Dento-Cranial Complex and lowered migraine pain was seen in all patients observed in test groups. Excess force generations and force overloads in the Dento-Cranial Complex were clearly demonstrated to be the cause of physical force trauma, cranial inflammation and migraine pain in all of the forty-five test group patients.

Physical force trauma is well known to be an underlying cause of inflammation and pain. Migraine pain relief seen after dental arch and chiropractic cranial adjustments done in the same time period were seen as a result of lower force generations and the associated force transfers that must occur according to universal laws of physics. This lowering of force generations, along with aligning force vectors in the Dento-Cranial Complex by altering hard tissue areas of contacts, with *Area* and *Pressure* being key factors used in mathematical calculations in force formulas utilized and applied in this migraine project.

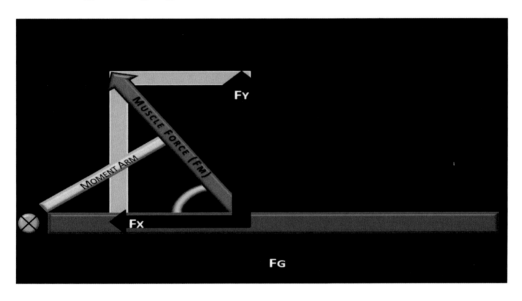

Components of Muscle Contraction and Force Transmission

Lowering of biomechanical force generations directly correlated with migraine pain relief in patients forty-five times in a row after alterations in hard tissues in dental arches and cranial bones were performed, leading to conclusions of DCFD being the cause of migraine pain in these patients, as relief of migraine pain was achieved soon after reduction of force loads and correction of vectors in this area of concentrated anatomy. The same is seen after Botox injections that reduce muscle contractions and contractile pressure gradients by partially paralyzing muscle fibers. Botox injections, however, do not produce a long-term solution such as seen after alterations in hard tissues.

Mathematics helped us to reliably ascertain this conclusion and confirm force magnitudes as a source of force overloads in this migraine project that contribute to physical force overload trauma that in turn causes migraine pain. Patterns of abnormally large contact areas of hard tissues were seen and measured in test groups and used to quantify force magnitudes being generated in the Dento-Cranial Complex prior to the corrective regimen being delivered. The use of the pure science of mathematics helped to guide the investigative process. This doctors group knew that as force loads increase, that their transfer, or dissipation must also occur according to universal laws of physics.

The force overload phenomenon labeled DCFD and described in detail by the doctor's group was seen as a cause of continuous physical force trauma. Continuous physical force trauma typically leads to physiologic response of cellular inflammation that causes pain, swelling, and heat generation to occur. DCFD describes a source of physical force trauma that is a clear cause of inflammation in the head and cranium. The group was successful in duplicating a corrective biofunctional process that produced migraine pain relief in test groups of patients who suffered from chronic headaches or migraines. Excess biomechanical forces that comprise DCFD were undeniably at the core of clinical symptoms of migraine pain in patients corrected, as relief rapidly ensued after biofunctional corrections.

The corrective process for DCFD initially discovered was based upon relief of symptoms caused by force overloads. Further conclusions reached were based on logic as well as on pure science of mathematics and physics Dento-Cranial Force Disorder (DCFD) has been proven using the scientific method of testing and duplication to be a source of physical force trauma that causes traumatic inflammation and migraine pain. Correction of this disorder repeatedly led to drastic relief of chronic headache pain on all forty-five patients in a row in initial test group observed, which was then used on more.

"Science is the acceptance of what works and the rejection of what does not. That needs more courage than we might think"

Jacob Bronowski

CHAPTER 2
INVISIBLE FORCES, HEAT &
INFLAMMATION

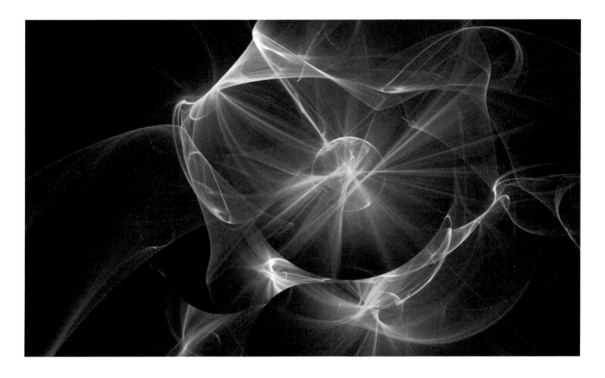

Invisible Forces that we cannot see... Abound

When a force occurs in nature, an equal and opposite force or reaction is also generated. These forces must somehow be dissipated. This is a well-known concept in science. Excess biomechanical force mechanics appear to develop from muscles compressing bone and hard dental structures together, which in turn translate into pressure-force gradients from the biomechanics in the Dento-Cranial Complex. According to universal laws of mathematics and physics, forces must be dissipated or transferred. Dissipation of forces generated in the Dento-Cranial Complex of muscles and bones occurs throughout the hard and soft tissues in this area of concentrated anatomy. A doctors cooperative group recognized that force generations and their transfer mechanics in the head were altered by dental and chiropractic adjustments that directly related to reduced migraine pain observed in patients, which led to investigation and in-depth analysis of force types and their transfers in the Dento-Cranial complex.

Normal dissipation of forces that are within biological tolerances, are simply absorbed by tissues, just as a knee joint and surrounding bones and muscles of the legs absorb and transfer mechanical loads and physical shock from walking or running. Forces created by muscle contractions cause forward movement of our body mass, and excess forces dissipate by flexible muscle fibers and bone flexure, just like springs in an automobile suspension function. When there is force overload or "out of balance force" a strain or injury occurs, which typically creates traumatic inflammation accompanied by swelling and pain. In the case of the head and cranium, there is no escape valve for excess pressure created by force overloads that occur daily in the Dento-Cranial Complex, as the head and brain are encased in a closed system inside the bony skull covering. Excess forces that cannot be absorbed by the surrounding tissues are considered to be in "excess of biological tolerances" and would logically and predictably lead to inflammation and pain inside this closed system of the cranium.

The chiropractor in the group introduced an infrared heat detection thermography device that he had been using on his patients to see heat patterns. These thermoscans allowed heat patterns indicative of inflammation to be seen like a visual thermometer. He had used this protocol on the experimental female dentist patient before starting his treatments, which showed significant cranial heat patterns before the biofunctional regimen was delivered by him, the dentist, and the osteopathic medical doctor. The group also began using this heat measuring technology with new test patients before delivery of the biofunctional corrective regimen that was being evaluated. This technology showed higher heat patterns in cranial areas scanned before biofunctional treatments were delivered, and lower heat after.

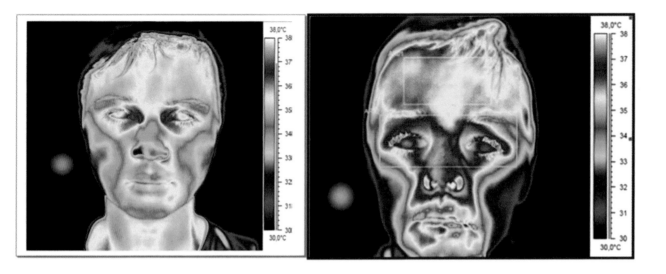

Thermographic Scans showing higher heat patterns on Right

Trauma and Inflammation

It is well known that force overloads in the body can lead to inflammation and pain, and further that heat is a telltale sign of inflammation. The group was looking for a way to pinpoint where traumatic force trauma was coming from in the context of head anatomy in an effort to help explore techniques to alter and correct force transmissions in the Dento-Cranial Complex that would help relieve migraine pain.

The group discussed how trauma causes inflammatory responses that start at the cellular level, causing chemicals to be released that initiate physiologic actions to occur that induce swelling and heat to occur in tissues. Inflammation leads to pain, with associated heat patterns that are visible using thermography scans.

It was further known that reduction of heat is a sign of resolution of inflammation. Deductive reasoning told us that if force overloads were the cause of an inflammatory response and if lowering of force loads and transfers led to reduction in heat generation and pain in the same tissues, then

27

a direct cause and effect relationship existed. This is exactly what was seen in patient groups who suffered from chronic migraine pain.

Resolution of migraine pain and concurrent reduction of head-heat patterns were repeatedly seen in test groups of patients treated with the biofunctional corrective regimen, with reduction in head- heat patterns observed within days of the corrective regimen being instituted. The doctors' group was now convinced that traumatic force overloads were the etiology of migraine pain in all of the patients observed, as the corrective regimen caused complete or near complete resolution of symptoms in all patients who received the corrective processes that was discovered and refined.

Reduction of head-heat patterns seen after corrective procedures using infrared thermoscans added further validation of the resolution of inflammation, as heat is one of the pathognomonic or telltale signs of inflammation.

"If I have seen further, it is by standing on the shoulders of Giants"

Isaac Newton

CHAPTER 3
WHY BIOFUNCTIONAL CORRECTIONS ARE SO SUCCESSFUL

This collaboration of doctors demonstrated that a corrective regimen that altered and corrected force magnitudes and their vectors in the jaws and cranial structures was responsible for migraine relief seen in the patient groups observed. This group of doctors perfected a regimen and duplicated results in an initial test group of forty-five patients that produced long-term resolution of migraine pain in all of these patients.

The doctors group considered the results observed to be clear cause and effect of inflammation and migraine pain caused by traumatic force overloads of DCFD. They believed their findings to be monumental with the potential to benefit countless other people who suffer with chronic migraine pain using the procedures and corrective regimen they discovered and refined.

Heavy compressive and pressure forces generated in the Dento-Cranial Complex have not previously been generally recognized as a source of head trauma that induces inflammation that causes migraines. One reason may be that these forces themselves are invisible, just as gravity is invisible. Another reason is that parameters such as contacting areas of hard tissues and muscular pressure generations that contribute to increased force magnitudes are difficult to visualize in the head, dental arches, and cranial bones.

Scenarios seen to date indicate that even slight changes in contact areas of hard tissues such as dental enamel in back teeth for example, can cause drastic changes in force generations. Enamel contact areas of back teeth in dental arches serve as force point-transfer areas to other structures higher up that jaw bones and powerful muscle groups press together hundreds of times daily. This squeezing together of structures can create significant compressive and pressure force generations that lead to force overloads.

The forces generated in the Dento-Cranial Complex logically travel up and into the head into the cranium, and when they are in excess of biologic tolerances of surrounding tissues to absorb, they induce traumatic inflammation and often migraine pain. Most people with migraine headache pain go to medical providers to seek medication to help alleviate this pain. However, the underlying cause of DCFD and Dento-Cranial force overloads discussed in this publication is something that medical providers are mostly not yet aware, and simply cannot see. Many dentists who may be able to detect the dental component are not trained in the specific multidisciplinary corrective realignment regimen that was discovered that includes chiropractic manipulations and realignments coordinated with dental procedures to help resolve the source of force overload induced traumatic inflammation that appears to be the cause of most migraine pain.

Most non-medical practitioners are also reluctant to get involved in the topic of "Migraine" as this has historically been considered to be solely a medical issue; however, the force overloads described in this publication start in the jaws and dental arches that can best be recognized by a specially trained dental-chiropractic team.

Use of Botox in medical practice has been successful in relieving migraine pain by lessening muscle contraction pressure, which further validates the force overload theory of etiology. Botox functions by partially paralyzing muscle fibers, which reduces pressure generations of muscles. Reducing muscle pressure generations via partial paralysis of muscle fibers reduces overall force generations in the Dento-Cranial Complex that are seen in mathematical conclusions when modified downward by reducing pressure numerators in force formulas. This group discovered that specific adjustments to hard tissues connecting and contacting areas in the Dento

Cranial Complex including teeth, dental arches, and cranial bones also lowered force generations in the Dento-Cranial Complex according to known mathematical formulas, with mathematics being a pure science that lacks speculation. In other words, our findings of lower force generations in the Dento-Cranial Complex after specific alterations were made was supported by mathematical calculations and conclusions using known force formulas.

Lasting reductions of force generations achieved in the dento-cranial complex using the corrective regimen developed by this group reduced compression and pressure force generations which are the prominent components of Dento-Cranial Force Disorder (DCFD). The biofunctional corrective regimen discovered and perfected achieves lowered force generations in the Dento-Cranial Complex without need for injections of Botox-paralyzing agent into muscles in the head and facial areas.

Long-term success in eliminating painful migraine episodes after delivery of dental and chiropractic corrective regimen has been observed for several years as of this writing. There has been minimal need for follow up refinement in the years following corrective regimens being completed, which is typically is accomplished over a one -to-two-week period on average. The refined biofunctional regimen is also performed in a particular sequence to maximize long-term resolution of excess force generations associated with chronic migraine pain. The combined regimen that was refined over time is drug free and non-invasive.

The discovery of this Force Overload Disorder and refinement of a corrective regimen to correct and lower force generations and transfers has helped hundreds of patients to date to be relieved of chronic migraine pain at such a high success rate indicating that this discovery is of extreme significance beyond any past known approaches.

The doctors group thought how significant their findings could be for millions of people in need of long-term migraine pain relief. They discussed

31

a similarity to the incidental discovery of penicillin in 1928 when Dr. Alexander Fleming accidentally dropped breadcrumbs into a petri dish in his lab in London that led to his incidental discovery of penicillin, which was not put into widespread use until 1940. Force overloads produced in the Dento-Cranial Complex have clearly been demonstrated to be a cause of migraine pain caused by force overloads that start in the jaw and dental complex and propagate and transfer up into the head and cranium. This realization along with the corrective remedy discovered and described in this book was also incidentally discovered.

All patients who took part in round one of this migraine project responded with near or complete resolution of chronic migraine pain within two weeks or less after delivery of the corrective regimen, demonstrating a direct correlation of Dento-Cranial Force Disorder (DCFD) to migraine pain.

Abnormally large contact areas of hard tissues in the Dento-Cranial Complex were seen in all patients exhibiting DCFD, including teeth, dental arches, and cranial bone connections called sutures. Increased contact areas contributing to higher force generations and abnormal transmissions were observed to increase over time in many people. Higher forces were observed in patient populations to develop over time from causes such as wear of hard surfaces against each other increasing contact areas as well as arch form deviations that are genetically influenced and contribute to force overload mechanics by their design, as well as other related bone morphology.

Abnormal sizes and shape of hard tissues in the Dento-Cranial Complex and the way they interconnect was seen as influential in force mechanics and related force overloads that collectively comprises this disorder that appears causative of most migraine pain syndromes. The highest prevalence of this disorder was observed to be in females who had past orthodontic treatment which alters dental arch forms and interdigitation of dental units leading to abnormal force mechanics and increased force generations.

Force overloads and concurrent larger parameters were observed in hundreds of patients to date that contribute to DCFD that appears to be prevalent in the population. All test groups of patients observed who were relieved of migraine pain exhibited large contact areas and /or high muscle pressure generations which combine to generate force overloads characteristic of DCFD.

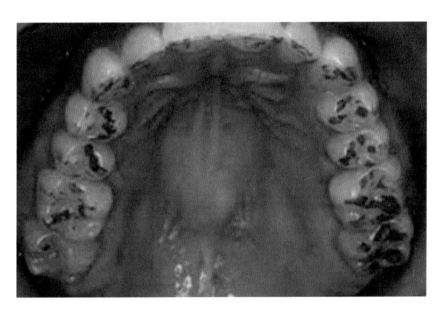

Large Bite Contact Areas in a dental arch that contribute to Excess Force Generations

All patients observed in test groups presenting with migraine history also exhibited DCFD in conjunction with migraine pain syndromes. These same groups also experienced rapid resolution of migraine pain after a biofunctional corrective regimen was employed. It was further demonstrated with mathematical certainty that this underlying force overload disorder is a very common with people who suffer migraine head pain, and further that it is a correctable to effect reduction of force overloads and transmissions in the Dento-Cranial Complex that provided long-term relief of migraine pain. Force loads calculated were observed to be significantly higher prior to corrective regimen delivery and drastically less after the corrective regimen, which is exactly what was expected from mathematical analysis before corrections.

Higher forces were seen to cause traumatic inflammation and pain that resolved when force magnitudes were reduced, and vectors of transmission corrected. Mathematical calculations of forces generated could now be seen on paper before and after corrective regimens were delivered.

Resolution of head pain also correlated with lowered force generations seen after the corrective regimen. In addition, lowered head-heat patterns seen on thermal scans introduced by the chiropractor were also seen within days after the corrective regimen was initiated.

This doctors group appears to have perfected a biofunctional corrective process that successfully lowers force generations and abnormal vectors of transmission that occur constantly in the Dento-Cranial Complex that transmit to the head and cranium that are intertwined in a puzzle of chronic migraine pain.

The group determined how to use mathematical force formulas and numerical calculations to relatively quantify excess forces before correction and determine lower force loads expected after corrections…. the same forces that were previously postulated to cause chronic migraine pain. Reduced heat signatures seen on thermography scans after the corrective regimen provided validation of lowered heat generation indicating resolution of inflammation, which all doctors in this group felt was extremely significant in validating the resolution of inflammation. Mathematics provided guidance and validation using pure science, which lacks speculation. The math relating to force loads helped the group better understand why such dramatic clinical resolutions of head pain were being seen after traumatic force overloads that had caused inflammation and pain were lessened.

All in the group were aware that powerful muscle groups connect jaws to each other and squeeze lower and upper units together with the most powerful muscle groups per unit area in the human body, collectively known as muscles of mastication. These are primarily the Masseter and Temporalis muscle groups. Masseter muscles are known to be capable of creating in excess of 1,000 pounds per square inch of compressive force generations. The mathematics utilized by the doctors group helped them to see excessive force loads as a source of trauma that can induce traumatic inflammation and pain in the head and cranium.

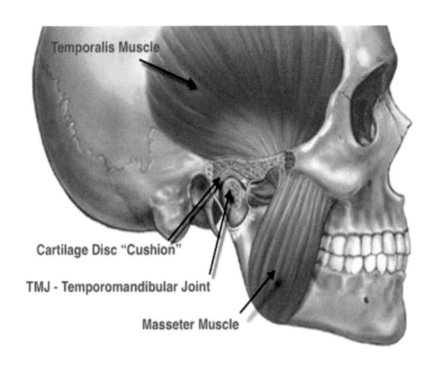

Powerful muscles in the human body attach upper and lower jaw bones to the cranium are capable of Contractile Forces in excess of 1,000 pounds per square inch.

Powerful jaw muscles squeeze the hard tissues of teeth and jaw bones together, creating compressive and pressure forces in the head. These forces create pressure waves of sorts that travel upwards into the head. This puts pressure on the thin, soft tissue covering of the brain under the skull called the meninges that is loaded with sensory nerves. When this pressure phenomenon occurs, it may be visualized as a blown-up balloon in a bottle squeezing against the outside edges, only in the head, pressure forces pressing outward against the thin, soft tissue covering of the brain called meninges, which is less than 1-millimeter thick and concentrated with sensory nerves. This would logically cause inflammation from traumatic pressure forces occurring from the inside pressing out. Pressure such as this would be sufficient to stimulate head pain that can be perceived as emanating from different areas.

"Every new body of discovery is mathematical in form, because there is no other guidance we can have"

Charles Darwin

CHAPTER 4
DISPELLING HISTORICAL DOGMA

"Migraine", or chronic headache syndrome, has historically been diagnosed solely on frequency of occurrence and severity alone. No other tests are typically employed, and no other confirming scientific tests, instruments, or apparatus have been used to confirm any aspect of this disorder. No specific cause has ever been identified, with the exception of the rare instances of internal head tumors that cause head pain from an abnormal internal growth. Mainstream therapy for migraines has focused primarily on drugs to mask pain or reduce the inflammatory process. Most realize that this treats *symptoms* and not a *cause*. Considering findings presented herein, this paradigm should begin to be reconsidered.

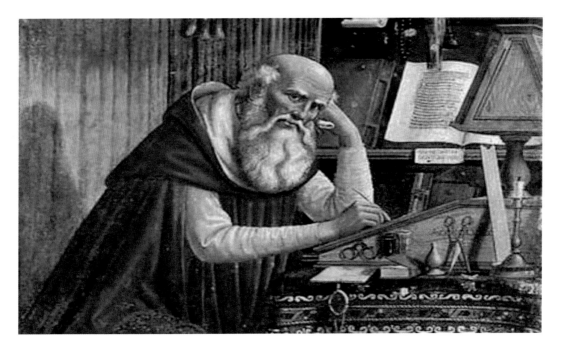

We have been looking for answers and solutions to chronic headaches since the time of Hippocrates.

It is interesting to note that the meninges soft tissue covering of the brain is the only area in the brain that contains sensory nerve fibers that transmit pain. The symptoms discussed and perceived by people who suffer migraine pain are all characteristic of inflammation of the meninges, the part of the brain that does possess the ability to perceive pain. Since the only pain receptors in the brain are in the meninges soft tissue covering envelope around the brain, underneath the skull bone, surgery can actually be performed on the brain and the patient does not feel pain. Although the brain does not sense pain directly, it is surrounded by membranes, blood vessels and muscles in the meninges that do contain sensory nerves that perceive and transmit pain.

Since the time of Hippocrates theories have abounded that postulate that etiology of chronic, repetitive moderate to severe headaches known as Migraines today, and the "Prodromal" or precursor symptoms, are caused by swollen intracranial blood vessels. This theory began nearly 2,000 years ago and remains center point to this day. The 20th century brought forth new imaging techniques that allowed for visualization of these swollen blood vessels, lending credibility to this theory.

But...what is causing the inflammation in the first place? The authors' conclusions are that inflammation in the head and cranium appear very clearly to be caused by Dento-Cranial force overloads, as surely as if you were bonking yourself with a small hammer on the side of your head several hundred times a day. Historically, the origin of the pain in a migraine headache has not been fully understood. After this publication, hopefully a new understanding will ensue for many. Dento-Cranial Force Theory should soon dispel past theories and hypotheses that have postulated an "Inflammatory Process of Unknown Etiology".

"Preconceived ideas are like searchlights which illuminate the path of experimenter and serve him as a guide to interrogate nature. They become a danger only if he transforms them into fixed ideas - this is why I should like to see these profound words inscribed on the threshold of all the temples of science: "The greatest derangement of the mind is to believe in something because one wishes it to be so"

Louis Pasteur

CHAPTER 5
TRIGGERS VS. CAUSE

This group observed that many people who suffer from migraines believe that triggers such as weather changes, bright lights, loud noises, sugar, alcohol, certain spices, or estrogen level changes in females, somehow cause migraines. None of these "triggers" have ever been shown to be a direct cause of inflammation. Triggers are precipitating factors that may stimulate a process, but are not a cause, which is vastly different. The underlying cause of pain and swelling in the human body is inflammation.

Traumatic Force overloads made much more sense to all of us as a true etiologic cause of headache pain, especially in light of the near 100% success that was witnessed in alleviating pain in our patient groups after reduction and correction of abnormal force generations and transfers were effected via biofunctional corrections.

Force overloads of DCFD observed in the Dento-Cranial Complex are capable of inducing traumatic inflammation in the head and cranium on an ongoing basis, which would allow triggers to easily induce painful episode in a system already inflamed, just like a sprained ankle that you can walk on but cannot run on without inducing acute pain.

An analogy of low-level force overloads occurring repeatedly over time also thought of was "the hammer on the head analogy" where a patient hits the side of their head several hundred times a day with a small round tipper ball peen hammer. It may not hurt for a while, but after several hundred blows, especially when occurring repeatedly over time, would absolutely lead to a low-level state of inflammation and pain in the head. In a state of constant low-level inflammation, the slightest trigger could easily stimulate an "over the cliff" painful episode, the same as seen when trying to run on an inflamed and tender sprained ankle. Force overloads from DCFD observed would have the same effect as this hammer on the head. They can cause sub-clinical trauma and inflammation on an ongoing basis, leading to either outright pain or "sensitive brain syndrome," where just like with a sprained ankle, small overloads can induce painful episodes.

Considering the findings presented herein, theories that postulate etiology of chronic headaches and precursor and or "Prodromal" symptoms to be caused by swollen intracranial blood vessels, should consider DCFD as a primary cause of the inflammation that lead to swollen vessels that may stem from traumatic force overloads.

The "Vasodilation Theory" or swollen blood vessels that are believed to cause the pain of migraine headaches is something the authors also subscribe to in part, but what has eluded scientists and health care providers for centuries until now is:

What causes the cranial inflammation that causes migraine pain?

There now appears to be a logical answer.

The force overload phenomena discovered and labeled "DCFD" is a logical cause of traumatic force induced inflammation and appears with mathematical certainty to be the overwhelming cause of chronic headaches, including those labeled migraines, as surely as if you would induce inflammation and pain from hitting yourself on the side of the head hundreds of times daily with that small round tipped hammer. Prior to this publication, "Migraine Headaches" have remained solely a symptom-based diagnosis, i.e., by frequency and severity only, not founded on any serologic fluid or other measurable test, either biological or electronic.

Other past theories have postulated many other different possible causes, yet none appear to have a logical basis as to the etiology of inflammation in the head and cranium that directly contributes to migraine pain; with inflammation being the underlying physiologic response to trauma that leads to swelling and pain in the human body. Theories such as "chemical messengers going astray" or nebulous brain stem disorders lack any verifiable scientific basis and have not been demonstrated or proven by any scientific means to date.

These postulations just have not made sense to the authors. Extensive publications in recent medical literature state that "Sterile Cranial Inflammation" appears to contribute to migraine head pain, meaning that cranial inflammation is present that is not caused by any biologic or viral invader. Sterile cranial inflammation of non-biologic origin is exactly what would be expected from force overloads presented herein.

Prior to this publication, no plausible explanation or scientific finding has been brought forth as to what causes cranial inflammation and migraine pain to occur in the first place. DCFD is now seen as being responsible for excess force generation in the head and cranium that is a logical cause of traumatic inflammation that can cause migraine head pain. This condition, when corrected, repeatedly produced total or near total migraine headache pain resolution along with reduced head-heat signatures seen on infra-red thermogram images occurring shortly after delivery of corrective regimen.

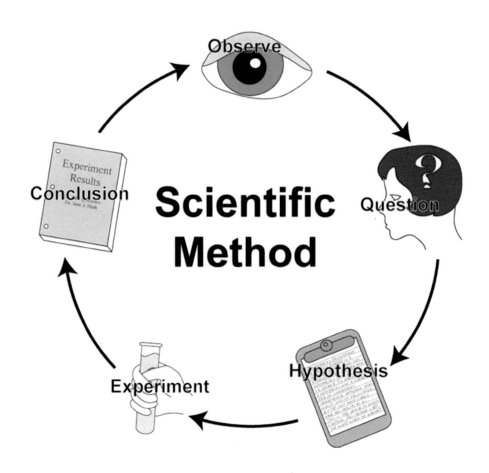

The "Scientific Method" diagrammed above, states that when an observation is made, from which a hypothesis is derived, one should formulate the hypothesis, quantify, or explain it, test it, identify results, then repeat to see if the same result occurs. Our conclusions followed this model showing the same results forty-five times in a row.

As DCFD becomes more widely known and more patients are successfully treated, it is likely to become known as the primary cause of chronic headaches or migraines, as staggering success rates seen in hundreds of patients to date indicate. Some extremely severe and chronic cases observed took longer to resolve, but all patients treated to date demonstrated reductions in severity and frequency of painful episodes within days after the corrective regimen was instituted, with near or complete resolution within weeks. The discovery of this hidden etiology and corrective regimen has the clear potential to be a game changer for millions of people in need of relief from this age-old malady.

As findings of this doctor's group were shared with peer groups, an ever-greater combined experience and awareness formed as the think tank grew to include more doctors from medical, osteopathic, dental implant specialists, chiropractors, and PhD's in engineering and biomechanics, many who contributed to this publication and to the *"Migraines Final Chapter"* full length book to follow.

"The world as we have created it is a process of our thinking. It cannot be changed without changing our thinking."

Albert Einstein

CHAPTER 6
WHY ARE WOMEN MORE AFFECTED?

When the logic of DCFD is embraced, the rationale of why women are more affected becomes quite sensible and understandable. The most plausible and logical explanation is that women's bones and tissues are physiologically softer and thus more sensitive to force overloads. Smaller amounts of trauma in women, whatever the source, can cause a more pronounced inflammation, greater damage, and greater pain than in men.

Previous theories of why women are more affected with chronic headache syndrome or migraines have been postulated in part to be caused by systemic estrogen imbalances, as estrogen does have an effect on contraction and relaxation of vessels; however, it appears that DCFD contributes to constant states of head and cranial inflammation of varied degrees from traumatic force overloads, which would logically allow minor triggering events to induce painful episodes.

Estrogen involvement in regulation of bone metabolism also appears to be a pertinent aspect of "The Estrogen Connection" and a logical reason as to *WHY* women are more affected. Women's bones are softer and smaller, whereas men's bones are larger and more robust. Weaker structures in the body, wherever they are located, logically translate into less ability to withstand stress of any kind.

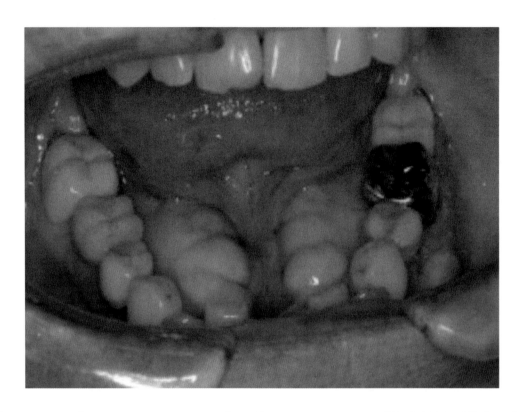

Bone hypertrophy , an overgrowth phenomenon called "Tori" in the lower arch of a 40-year-old male from force overloads

Bone hypertrophy is overgrowth seen in many patients' mouths, with greater prevalence in men. This bone enlargement occurs in response force overloads, the same as seen in long bones from weightlifting in response to force loads placed upon bones in areas subjected to extra force loads. The male patient seen above had no headaches but needed several crowns for fractured teeth. This bone overgrowth occurs less frequently in females; however, females experience more chronic headaches from the same underlying etiology of this bone overgrowth pictured above: Force Overloads!

Observations of dentists in the group over many years were that women react to increased forces with more headaches while men tend to wear down or crack teeth more than seen in females. Excess clinching or grinding of teeth was observed by this group to be less tolerated by women, before a pain responses occurs. It appears that women are simply less able to withstand

and dissipate constant, excessive compressive forces generated in the Dento-Cranial Complex than men.

Altered estrogen levels in women have been correlated to increased incidence of migraine pain or chronic headache syndrome; however, altered estrogen levels appear to be a predisposing factor or a trigger, not a predominate cause. Since migraine headaches are much more prevalent in females, there appears to be a historical lack of clarity as to the estrogen connection hypothesis.

Our group observed that patients who were corrected and relieved of migraine pain were no longer susceptible to previous triggering events causing painful episodes. The topic of inflammation and hormone imbalance as well as physiology of why women are more affected than men is also discussed in great detail in the upcoming full length follow up book release of "*Migraines Final Chapter*".

"Nothing in life is to be feared; it is only to be understood"

Marie Curie

CHAPTER 7
WHY THE CAUSE & SOLUTION HAVE BEEN SO ELUSIVE?

Medical researchers and clinicians have historically looked for organic causes of migraines as such is the cognitive system and bias of medicine that has evolved since the time of Hippocrates. When an underlying cause is not organic in nature, research into non-drug therapy is not likely to be funded by traditional sources such as drug manufacturers. Sales of pharmaceuticals both over the counter and prescribed exceed seventy billion dollars annually in the USA alone. Now, there are a couple of surgical procedures to add into the mix such as counter stimulating devices that are being surgically implanted into foreheads to mask pain transmission from inflamed sensory nerves in the area where the ophthalmic branch of Trigeminal cranial nerve exits the skull by each eyebrow. Incidental discovery of reduced pain perception of migraines was first observed after plastic surgeries in this area. Trigeminal nerve which has three separate trunks or divisions, is the prime nerve pipeline for pain transmission in the head, including all jaw and dental pain.

Drugs that alter, change, or mask the inflammatory or pain transmission process continue to be a prime topic of research, always looking for more and improved variations. Many patients have reported that after receiving the corrective regimen discovered by this group that greatly lessened or completely ameliorated migraine pain, the need for daily medication was also greatly reduced or eliminated.

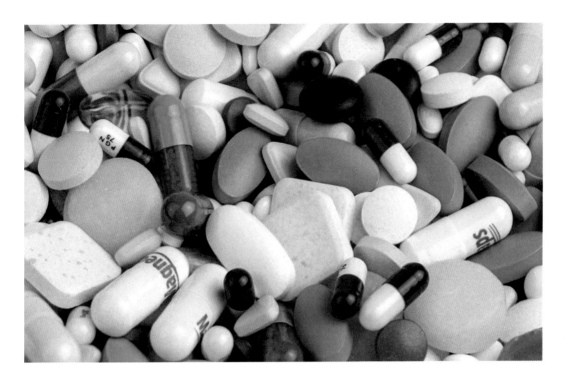

Drugs, the traditional approach treating symptoms, not the cause.

The educational process of medical schools has also focused on ways to manage pain of Chronic Headaches, or Migraines, which has been accepted as emanating from "Inflammation of Unknown Etiology" in a condition that has had "No Known Cause."

It appears to this authoring doctors' group that researchers and clinicians have been looking for an organic cause that simply does not exist. Dental Schools touch on chronic head pain from TMJ (temporomandibular joint dysfunction) as a syndrome that has chronic headaches in part, but the overall category of chronic headaches has for the most part, succumbed to an accepted mantra that "there is no known cure," and that alleviation of pain symptoms has been accepted to be the domain of medical practitioners. Our findings shed new light on that mantra.

Contributing to the historical elusive handle on etiology of "Sterile Cranial Inflammation" believed by many to be the underlying cause of pain of migraine, is a chronic disconnect that has also existed between medical and dental science and practice. This disconnect is also apparent for chiropractic and medical science and practice. Some dental practitioners in the past have found that using various orthopedic jaw devices, appliances, or other devices to alter dental bite forces or occlusion schemes in the past have produced reductions in headache pain. This included many patients that were also suffering from temporomandibular joint dysfunction or related dental bite imbalances. However, whenever the topic of "migraine" came up, dentists would most often punt the ball back to medical practitioners for pain management and overall medical analysis. This is likely due in part also to the small percentage of patients that developed some sort of growth inside their brain such as a tumor, a cyst, or a fluid filled sac, and since rare abnormal growths do occur, it has influenced most dental and chiropractic practitioners away from trying to help for fear of missing that one in a million, and somehow being held liable. In essence, this scares most away.

Further to this, the corrective regimen discovered and refined is very technique specific, multifaceted, and complex. If not property performed, increased force generations could be created that may make a bad situation even worse. Most dentists have also been reluctant to be involved in "treatment of migraines" for fear of prosecution by regulatory boards for practicing medicine without a license, in addition to the possibility of somehow being responsible for rare brain tumors that do occur.

All the above concerns contribute to most dentists leaving chronic headaches or migraines to the domain of medical practice, as illogical as that has been found to be when considering contributions that some dental providers and appliances and have provided. Historically if a person has migraines or a family history of migraines, a medical doctor trained in treating headaches, such as a neurologist, typically diagnoses migraines based primarily on history and symptoms. Considering nearly 40-million people in the United Stated alone are estimated to suffer chronic headache pain and as many as one billion people worldwide, or approximately 15% of the population, it would seem help from any source would be welcomed.

A World Center for Migraine Relief is underway near the international border of San Diego, California where the initial group has participated in various teaching programs for other doctors as well as helping many in need from the international community.

"Divine is the task to relieve pain"

Hippocrates

CONCLUSIONS

Dento-Cranial Force Disorder (DCFD) should soon predominate as a primary underlying etiologic cause of migraines or chronic headache syndrome. This authoring collaboration of doctors has grown to include researchers in biomechanics and several other health care areas, all contributing specific knowledge and input to this migraine project.

All involved to date believe that previously unrecognized Dento- Cranial Force Disorder (DCFD) is likely to be the primary etiology of most migraines in the population who suffer. It has been clinically proven to a mathematical certainty that DCFD causes migraine pain and that when this underlying disorder is corrected, migraine pain is greatly reduced or completely alleviated.

Prior to this publication, the actual etiology and cause of migraine pain has eluded the healing professions and scientific community since it was first recognized and described during the time of Hippocrates in ancient Greece.

This group discovered DCFD and identified specific parameters that effect force generations and their magnitudes in the Dento-Cranial Complex. They also determined how these forces transmit up into the head and cranium to cause inflammation and migraine pain. The factors that generate compressive and pressure forces in the Dento-Cranial Complex that start with muscle contractions, were identified, and measured. This included muscular contraction pressures and contacting areas of various hard tissues in the head including contact and load bearing areas in enamel transfer points of teeth and dental arches, and cranial bone plate connections above the upper jaws. All were seen to relate to force generations and their dissipations that in turn related to the overall puzzle that has been the migraine enigma.

54

Mathematics was used to help perfect a methodology to lower forces that is not speculative in any way. Corrective methodology successfully used in hundreds of patients to date drastically lowered or eliminated migraine pain in all who were biofunctionally corrected. Chiropractic alignment of skeletal bones also was integral to the process. Increased force generations seen in the Dento-Cranial Complex in hundreds of patients to date were significantly excessive in magnitude to cause excess force generations that can cause traumatic inflammation and head- pain known as migraine. Awareness that forces must be transferred or dissipated up into the head according to universal laws of physics, helped this group make sense of the age-old dilemma of migraines.

Mathematics helped to confirm our suspicions and guide us to a predictable corrective regimen that has been providing long-term relief. Force magnitudes were calculated using measurable parameters of pressure and contact areas identified, using known force calculation formulas, and were seen to be of sufficient magnitudes to constitute force overloads capable of inducing traumatic inflammation and pain from physical force load assaults in the head and cranium that occur hundreds of times daily.

It was clearly observed that when force magnitudes were lowered via biofunctional techniques discovered and refined by this group, that migraine pain dissolved away.

The high prevalence of DCFD observed in patient populations observed over time combined with high rate of success seen with patients relieved of chronic migraine pain after correction, led us to conclude that Dento-Cranial Force Disorder (DCFD) is likely to be the predominant cause of chronic headache syndromes or migraines in the population who suffer from these syndromes.

A corrective regime of primarily dental and chiropractic procedures performed in concert was incidentally discovered to relieve migraine pain that was determined to result from correction of force overloads in the Dento-Cranial Complex. The process discovered was investigated, thoroughly analyzed, refined, duplicated, and validated utilizing the scientific method of testing and analysis, as well as mathematics of force generations to validate findings of increased force magnitudes and their dissipation as the etiology of most migraine pain, as when they were reduced, migraine pain dissolved away.

The force overload phenomena discussed in this publication was seen to be the cause of chronic low-level states of inflammation in the head and cranium that resolved along with migraine pain after biofunctional corrections. This was validated in part by use of infra-red thermo scan imaging, as heat and pain are two of the three components of inflammation. Sterile cranial inflammation is seen extensively in medical publications as being present in people who suffer migraine headaches. Inflammation is known to be the cause of pain in the human system. Up until present time, the cause of this pain-inducing inflammation in the cranium had been unknown. Dento-Cranial Force Disorder was repeatedly and predictably demonstrated to be causative of trauma, inflammation, and migraine pain. DCFD further has been shown to be a correctable disorder using a biofunctional corrective regimen discussed in this book.

Once force overload induced traumatic inflammation was identified as the underlying cause of migraine pain, corrective procedures to reduce and correct force loads and their vectors were perfected over time that resolved underlying inflammation and associated migraine pain. Regenerative therapies and processes including hyperbaric oxygen therapy and occasional optional stem cell regenerative processes were subsequently added into the regimen that accentuated recovery and return to normalcy for many chronic migraine sufferers.

The biofunctional corrective regimen referenced in this publication has been successfully evaluated and proven in hundreds of patients to date at a

56

staggering rate of success in resolving chronic migraine pain. This success seen appears to speak for itself, as do the many patients who have been relieved of their migraine pain. Hundreds have been corrected and relieved of chronic migraine pain to date, which has merely scratched the surface of this malady that affects many millions. The rate of success seen in the high ninety percent range by this collaborative group to date indicates significance beyond any other modality previously seen with a potential to help provide a drug free, non-invasive, and painless avenue to provide lasting relief of chronic headache or migraine pain for the many who suffer.

The information presented in this book should serve as a beacon of hope and provide a path to the corrective methodology of this force overload cause of migraine pain. The authoring group has seen so many people's lives restored to normal again from this process. It appears that this etiology and corrective approach should help the majority of people who suffer from chronic headache syndromes including those labeled migraine.

It is hoped that you, the reader, see the logic that came about from our findings presented, and that it serves as a pathway to long-term recovery from chronic migraine pain.   Details of World Centers for Migraine Relief will be available online at

www.worldmigraine.com

"The nobelest pleasure is the joy of understanding"

-Leonardo da Vinci

Dear Dr. Mansueto,

Thank you so much for saving me from the torturous headaches and earaches that I suffered from for so long. I did not realize that a dentist and chiropractor could improve someone's life so much. After the corrections you did for me, not only do I smile a lot these days, but my entire outlook and attitude on life are much improved...a literal life changing attitude adjustment! I am letting all my friends and clients know of the wonderful gift of pain relief that you have given me.

Sincerely yours,
Rosalind Novitsky,
Hair stylist, San Diego

Dear Doctor Mansueto,

I just want to thank you for releasing me from my previous life. I am 28 years old and for the last 15 years I have suffered from severe and frequent migraines, which interfere with my everyday life in the most extreme way. I couldn't find peace. Well, after your treatments I finally can!

It turns out that my migraines were a result of some kind of pressure being produced in my jaws that went upward. I attended your clinic several times over a period of a few weeks, and it changed my life. No pain was involved. Thanks to you, now I hardly ever have migraines.

Sincerely,
Karen Landau, Imperial Beach, CA

Dear Doctor Mansueto,

A year ago, my wife Karen was suffering from severe migraines on a daily basis, which interfered with our normal life. When I heard of your treatment approach, we decided to give it a shot.

After only four visits, we saw a difference. My wife did not have a migraine every day, but every other day…and it got better and better every day.

Today, my wife almost does not suffer from any migraines at all. I can only thank your doctor's group for changing our lives for the best.

Best regards,

Alan Landau, paralegal, Phoenix, AZ

Dear Dr. Mansueto,

As you probably recall, you treated me for chronic headaches more than two years ago. Although this "24 month follow up report" is a little later than promised, I'm happy to report that the therapy approach provided (you referred to it as adjustment in force mechanics per unit area" or something along those lines) continues to be completely successful and I've been headache free since that time.

I'm not sure whether you recall, but I first experienced these migraine-like headaches when I was 18 years old or so and continued to suffer with them on a regular basis for more than 30 years despite taking several recommended medications. Nothing seemed to work, until the adjustments your group performed for me significantly ameliorated the problem. Allow me to express my sincerest thanks to you and your staff.

Sincerely,
Gary M. Carter College Professor, Petaluma, CA

REFERENCES

Anatomy and physiology of headache. Bogduk N. Biomed Pharmacother. 1995; 49(10):435-45.

A preliminary report on hyperbaric oxygen in the relief of migraine headache D E Myers [1],
R A Myers Pub Med.gov National Library of Medicine
https://pubmed.ncbi.nlm.nih.gov/7775175/

Association between signs and symptoms of bruxism and presence of tori: a systematic review Eduardo Bertazzo-Silveira [1], Juliana Stuginski-Barbosa [2], André Luís Porporatti [3], Bruce Dick [4], Carlos Flores-Mir [5], Daniele Manfredini [6], Graziela De Luca Canto Clin Oral   Investig 2017 Dec;21(9):2789-2799. 2017 Feb 17.
        https://pubmed.ncbi.nlm.nih.gov/28213765/

Biomechanics of Cranio-Maxillofacial Trauma J Maxillofacial Oral Surg. 2012 Jun; 11(2): 224–
        230.Published online 2011 Oct 9. doi: 10.1007/s12663-011-0289-7

Biomechanics: the keystone of treatment planning in osseointegration. *Martha Bidez, Ph.D*
        December 1994 Dental Implantology Update 5(11):81-4

Botox: Cosmetic and medical uses   Hannah Nichols August 10, 2020,
        https://www.medicalnewstoday.com/articles/158647

Contemporary Implant Dentistry Carl Misch Mosby Publishing Third Edition 2008

The Fifth Cranial nerve in headaches The Journal of Headache and Pain 21, Article number: 65
        (2020) J. C. A. Edvinsson, A. Viganò,

Functional Occlusion, Peter Dawson, DDS, 2007, Mosby Elsevier Publishing

The Great Occlusion Fiasco Gene McCoy, DDS *J Oral Implantol* (2017) 43 (3): 167–168. https://doi.org/10.1563/aaid-joi-D-17-00083

Handbook of Mathematical Tables and Formulas by Richard Stevens Burington

How to Tell when Chronic Headaches have a Dental Cause: Functional occlusion in patients with chronic headaches: Interview with Jeri Coffey, DDS Jeri Coffey, DDS, Ross A. Hauser, MD, Nicole M. Baird, CHFP, & Doug R. Skinkis *Journal of Prolotherapy. 2010;2(3):447-453*

The Integrative Migraine Pain Alleviation through Chiropractic Therapy ,[a,b,*,1] C. Bernstein,[c,d,1] M. Kowalski,[d] J.P. Connor,[a] K. Osypiuk,[a] C.R. Long,[e] R. Vining,[e] E. Macklin,[f] and P.M. Rist[b] Contemp Clin Trials Commun. 2020 Mar; 17: 100531. Published online 2020 Jan 22. doi: 10.1016/j.conctc.2020.100531

The Integrative Migraine Pain Alleviation through Chiropractic Therapy (IMPACT) trial: Study rationale, design and intervention validation P.M. Wayne,[a,b,*,1] C. Bernstein,[c,d,1] M. Kowalski,[d] J.P. Connor,[a] K. Osypiuk,[a] C.R. Long,[e] R. Vining,[e] E. Macklin,[f] and P.M. Rist[b] https://www.ncbi.nlm.nih.gov/pmc/articles/PMC6997836/

Migraine and the trigeminovascular system—40 years and counting Messoud Ashina, Jakob Møller Hansen, Thien Phu Do, Agustin Melo-Carrillo, Rami Burstein, and Michael A Moskowitz National Library of Medicine https://www.ncbi.nlm.nih.gov/pmc/articles/PMC7164539/

Migraine — Current Understanding and Treatment Peter J. Goadsby, M.D., D.Sc., Richard B. Lipton, M.D., and Michel D. Ferrari, M.D., Ph.D. New Engl J Med 2002:

Migraine pain, meningeal inflammation, and mast cells, D Levy, 2009 https://link.springer.com › article

Modern Implant Dentistry, second edition Mosby Publishers, 1999, Carl E. Misch et al

MRIs for Headache and Migraine Diagnosis https://www.webmd.com/migrainesheadaches/making-diagnosis-mri

Medically Reviewed by Jennifer Robinson, MD Jan2022

Nerve Fibers Innervating the Cranial and Spinal Meninges: Morphology of Nerve Fiber

Terminals and Their Structural Integration MICROSCOPY RESEARCH AND TECHNIQUE 53:96–105 (2001) BRITTA FRICKE,* KARL HERMANN ANDRES,

AND MONIKA VON DÜRING Department of Neuroanatomy, Institute of Anatomy, Ruhr University, Bochum, Germany

Neurogenic inflammation and its role in migraine Epub 2018 Mar 22. Roshni
Ramachandran

https://pubmed.ncbi.nlm.nih.gov/29568973/ - affiliation-1 National Library of Medicine
National Center for Biotechnology Information
      https://pubmed.ncbi.nlm.nih.gov/29568973/

Neurogenic Inflammation: The Participant in Migraine and Recent Advancements in

Translational Research. Spekker E, Tanaka M, Szabó Á, Vécsei L.Biomedicines. 2021
      Dec 30;10(1):76.

Occlusion Confusion G McCoy Dental Research and Management

Edelweiss Publications May 2019 https://doi.org/10.33805/2572-6978.120

One Hundred Years of Migraine Research: Major Clinical and Scientific Observations
From
1910 to 2010 Peer C. Tfelt-Hansen MD, PhD,Peter J. Koehler MD, PhDFirst published:

26 April 2011 https://doi.org/10.1111/j.1526-4610.2011.01892.x

Pain and intramuscular release of algesic substances in the masseter muscle after
experimental   tooth-clenching exercises in healthy subjects. J Dawson
A,Ghafouri B,et al. Orofac
Pain 27 (4) 2013

Pathophysiology of migraine 2012 Aug Academy of Neurology
      https://www.ncbi.nlm.nih.gov/pmc/articles/PMC3444225/

Pathophysiology of Migraine Vol 75:365-391 Nov 26, 2012. Daniela Pietrobon[1,2] and
Michael   A. Moskowitz[3] [1]Department of Biomedical Sciences, University of Padova
and [2]CNR
Institute of Neuroscience, 35121 Padova, Italy
Pathophysiology of Migraine: A Disorder of Sensory Processing. Goadsby PJ, Holland
PR,   Martins-Oliveira M, Hoffmann J, Schankin C, Akerman S.Physiol Rev. 2017
      Apr;97(2):553-622. doi: 10.1152/physrev.00034.2015.PMID: 28179394
      https://www.ncbi.nlm.nih.gov/pmc/articles/PMC5539409/

The impact of spinal manipulation on migraine pain and disability: a systematic review
and
meta-analysis. Rist P.M., Hernandez A., Bernstein C *Headache.* 2019;59(4):532–
      542. [PMC free article] [PubMed] [Google Scholar]

Thermography for the Diagnosis of Acute Inflammation in the Paranasal Sinus
https://www.ncbi.nlm.nih.gov/pmc/articles/PMC6986953/ IAO International
Archives of Otorhinolaryngology 2020 Apr

The trigeminal nerve. Shankland WE 2nd. Part II: the ophthalmic division. Cranio.
2001Jan;19(1):8-12.

What are the causes of migraine headache? Updated: Oct 01, 2021, Jasvinder Chawla,
MD, MBA; Chief Editor: Helmi L Lutsep, MD https://www.medscape.com/ Medscape

Made in the USA
Las Vegas, NV
27 January 2024

84966793R00043